# Mayo Clinic
## Atlas of Immunofluorescence in Dermatology

### Patterns and Target Antigens

# Mayo Clinic
## Atlas of Immunofluorescence in Dermatology

## Patterns and Target Antigens

**Amer N. Kalaaji, MD**
Consultant
Department of Dermatology
Mayo Clinic
Assistant Professor of Dermatology
Mayo Clinic College of Medicine
Rochester, Minnesota

Co-author
**Marie Eleanore O. Nicolas, MD**
Immunodermatology Fellow
Mayo School of Graduate Medical Education
Mayo Clinic College of Medicine
Rochester, Minnesota
Presently Clinical Associate Professor
Section of Dermatology
University of the Philippines College of Medicine
Philippine General Hospital
Manila, Philippines

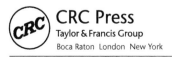

CRC Press
Taylor & Francis Group
Boca Raton London New York

CRC Press is an imprint of the
Taylor & Francis Group, an **informa** business

CRC Press
Taylor & Francis Group
6000 Broken Sound Parkway NW, Suite 300
Boca Raton, FL 33487-2742

First issued in paperback 2019

© 2006 by Taylor & Francis Group, LLC
CRC Press is an imprint of Taylor & Francis Group, an Informa business

No claim to original U.S. Government works

ISBN-13: 978-0-8493-7572-9 (hbk)
ISBN-13: 978-0-367-39097-6 (pbk)

Catalog record is available from the Library of Congress.

**Visit the Taylor & Francis Web site at**
**http://www.taylorandfrancis.com**

**and the CRC Press Web site at**
**http://www.crcpress.com**

# Preface

This atlas reviews the different immunofluorescence patterns for various dermatologic conditions through the use of photographs, brief descriptions, tables, and flowcharts. Some important aspects of immunofluorescence are described in the following paragraph.

Immunofluorescence testing is important for diagnosing immunobullous diseases, connective tissue diseases, and vasculitis. Direct immunofluorescence involves the overlay of fluorescein-conjugated antibodies (IgG, IgM, IgA), complement (C3), and fibrinogen onto frozen sections of tissue obtained from patients. Biopsy specimens for direct immunofluorescence in immunobullous disease should be taken from perilesional normal-appearing skin within a few millimeters of the edge of the blister. Obtaining a biopsy specimen from the blister or too close to the blister can result in a false-negative finding. This result is especially possible when dealing with mucosal surfaces because they are already prone to epithelial detachment. However, when a biopsy specimen is needed for diagnosis of connective tissue disease or vasculitis, a lesional biopsy is optimal.

Indirect immunofluorescence studies involve the detection of circulating autoantibodies in the patient's serum which target specific antigens in the patient's skin or mucosa. The technique for indirect immunofluorescence is helpful in immunobullous diseases. It involves incubating the patient's serum, which contains the autoantibodies, with frozen sections of epithelial substrate. The substrate is usually monkey esophagus, but pig esophagus also has been used. Rat bladder is used to rule out paraneoplastic pemphigus. After washing, fluoroscein-labeled animal anti-IgG conjugate against human immunoglobulin, such as IgG, is added. This fluoroscein-labeled animal conjugate binds to the patient's circulating IgG, which is already bound to the target antigen on the epithelial surface. Indirect immunofluorescence allows titration of the patient's serum to determine the highest titration yielding visible fluorescence. In cases of pemphigus, the titer of these autoantibodies correlates with disease activity.

This atlas systematically reviews the different immunofluorescence patterns found in immunodermatology for various immunobullous diseases, connective tissue diseases, vasculitis, and some miscellaneous conditions such as porphyria and lichenoid reactions. In addition, the direct and indirect immunofluorescence findings and the target antigens the autoantibodies bind to in various diseases are summarized in an easy-to-follow table.

I hope that this atlas will aid in understanding the different immunofluorescence patterns in many dermatology conditions. This atlas should be used by dermatologists, pathologists, residents, fellows, and medical students who obtain immunofluorescence results from patients. This atlas also will be a valuable resource for dermatology and pathology residents preparing for board examinations and is dedicated to all persons who have an interest in immunodermatology.

Immunodermatology has a long and rich tradition at Mayo Clinic, and I thank all my mentors in immunodermatology. You have inspired and taught, and I hope this atlas will help inspire the next generation of immunodermatologists. It has been a pleasure and a privilege to work with all my distinguished colleagues in dermatology at Mayo Clinic. Thank you for your teaching, mentoring, and friendship. I am grateful to my co-author and friend, Marie Nicolas, for her significant contributions to this atlas.

I especially thank my family for their love and support, which I cherish above all else. To my late father, I miss you and I thank you for your wisdom and continued inspiration.

Amer N. Kalaaji, MD

# Table of Contents

# Abbreviations

The following abbreviations are used throughout the book:

| | |
|---|---|
| **ANA** | antinuclear antibodies |
| **BMZ** | basement membrane zone |
| **BP** | bullous pemphigoid |
| **ICS** | intercellular space |
| **SSS** | salt-split skin |

# Linear Basement Membrane Zone Staining Pattern

A. Bullous Pemphigoid

B. Pemphigoid Gestationis (Herpes Gestationis)

C. Lichen Planus Pemphigoides

D. Mucous Membrane Pemphigoid

E. Bullous Lupus Erythematosus

F. Epidermolysis Bullosa Acquisita

G. Linear IgA Bullous Dermatosis

# Bullous Pemphigoid (BP)

**Clinical**

- Tense bullae on erythematous, urticarial, or normal skin
- Flexural predominance
- Elderly patients (typically older than 60 years)
- Generalized pruritus commonly associated
- Mucous membrane involvement (10%-40%)
- Absence of scarring (differs from cicatricial pemphigoid and epidermolysis bullosa acquisita)
- Variants
  - Localized BP to lower extremities (elderly)
  - Pemphigoid nodularis (prurigo nodularis with or without bullae)
  - Generalized pruritus and dermatitis
  - Urticarial pemphigoid
  - Tense acral bullae in infants and vulvar involvement in pre-pubertal girls

**Direct Immunofluorescence**

- Linear basement membrane zone (BMZ): IgG (90%)
- Linear BMZ: C3 (>90%, nearly all) (Fig. 1.1)

**Indirect Immunofluorescence**

- Linear BMZ: IgG on monkey esophagus substrate (circulating IgG antibody in 75% of cases; Fig. 1.2)
- Salt-split skin (SSS): epidermal pattern (Fig. 1.3)
- Occasionally combined epidermal-dermal pattern

**Target Antigens**

- BP230 (BPAG1)
- BP180 (BPAG2)
  - NC16A (immunodominant region of BP180)

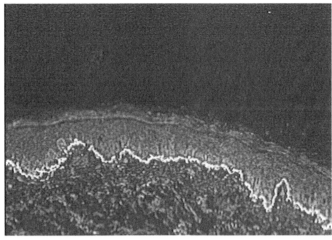

**Fig. 1.1** Linear BMZ: C3

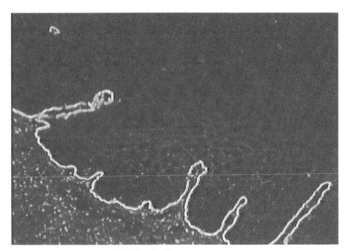

**Fig. 1.2** Linear BMZ: IgG

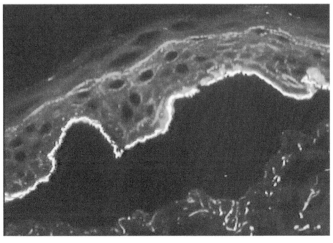

**Fig. 1.3** SSS: epidermal pattern

# Pemphigoid Gestationis (Herpes Gestationis)

| | |
|---|---|
| **Clinical** | ▪ Onset is usually during the second and third trimesters of pregnancy<br>▪ Can occur post partum (typically first 2-3 days post partum)<br>▪ Polymorphous skin eruption<br>  - Skin lesions range from urticarial papules and plaques to vesicles and bullae<br>▪ Typically spares mucous membranes<br>▪ Recurrences can develop with use of oral contraceptives<br>▪ Neonatal pemphigoid gestationis can occur from passive transfer of maternal IgG across the placenta |
| **Direct Immunofluorescence** | ▪ Linear BMZ: IgG (approximately 25% of cases)<br>▪ Linear BMZ: C3 (100% of cases, diagnostic) (Fig. 1.4) |
| **Indirect Immunofluorescence** | ▪ Linear BMZ: IgG (<25% of cases, does not correlate with disease activity)<br>▪ HG factor: 50% of cases<br>▪ SSS: epidermal pattern |
| **Target Antigens** | ▪ BP230 (BPAG1)<br>▪ BP180 (BPAG2) (most important)<br>  - NC16A (immunodominant region of BP180) |

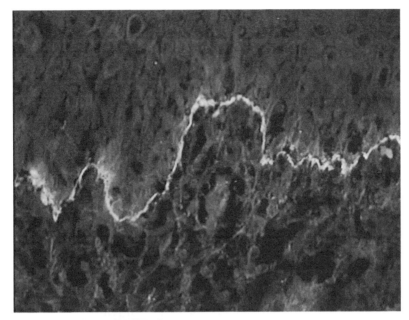

Fig. 1.4  Linear BMZ: C3

# Lichen Planus Pemphigoides

| | |
|---|---|
| **Clinical** | ■ Coexistence of lichen planus and bullous pemphigoid in the same patient<br>■ Bullae develop on normal-appearing skin away from lichen planus lesions and are due to circulating autoantibodies<br>■ In contrast, bullous lichen planus generally refers to bullae developing in lichen planus lesions as a result of the inflammatory infiltrate, epitope spreading, and no circulating antibodies |
| **Direct Immunofluorescence** | ■ Linear BMZ: IgG and C3 with changes of lichen planus (i.e., cytoid bodies with IgM, IgA, C3, and shaggy BMZ with fibrinogen) (Fig. 1.5) |
| **Indirect Immunofluorescence** | ■ Linear BMZ: IgG antibodies in 50% of patients<br>■ SSS: epidermal pattern |
| **Target Antigens** | ■ BP230 (BPAG1)<br>■ BP180 (BPAG2) (most important)<br>  - NC16A (immunodominant region of BP180) |

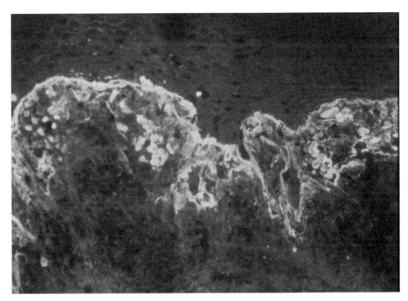

Fig. 1.5 Shaggy BMZ: fibrinogen

# Mucous Membrane Pemphigoid

**Clinical**
- Autoimmune subepithelial blistering disorder
- Predominantly involves mucosal surfaces with less skin involvement
- Chronic and recurring course
- Scarring tends to occur
- A "disease phenotype" shared by a heterogeneous group of diseases
- Severe mucosal involvement can result in blindness and laryngeal and esophageal stenosis

**Direct Immunofluorescence**
- Linear BMZ: IgG, C3, IgA

**Indirect Immunofluorescence**
- Linear BMZ: IgG in 15% to 20% of cases
- SSS: epidermal, dermal, or combined (Fig. 1.6)

**Target Antigens**
- BP230 (BPAG1)
- BP180 (BPAG2) (C-terminus and some NC16A)
- $\beta_4$ integrin subunit
- Laminin-5 (also called epiligrin, nicein, kalinin, BM600)
- Laminin-6
- Type VII collagen (290 kd)

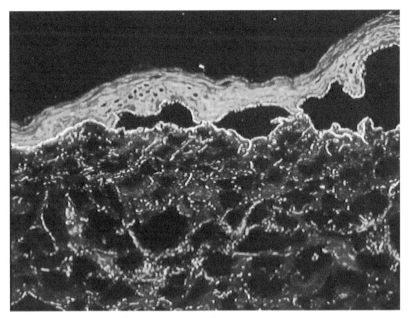

Fig. 1.6  SSS: combined epidermal-dermal pattern

# Bullous Lupus Erythematosus

**Clinical**

- Occurs typically in patients with systemic lupus erythematosus
- Photosensitivity is common
- Skin findings can include tense bullae, vesicles, urticarial vasculitis-like lesions, and cutaneous manifestations of systemic lupus erythematosus
- Skin findings typically have a photodistribution
- Scarring can occur
- Mucous membrane involvement (especially oral) can occur

**Direct Immunofluorescence**

- Linear BMZ: IgG and C3; IgM and IgA also (if perilesional biopsy of bullae) (Fig. 1.7)
- Granular BMZ: IgG, IgM, C3 (if lesional biopsy of malar rash or other cutaneous involvement of lupus) (Fig. 1.8)

**Indirect Immunofluorescence**

- Antinuclear antibodies (ANA)
- BMZ antibodies not detected on monkey esophagus but may be detected on SSS
- SSS: dermal pattern (IgG)

**Target Antigens**

- Type VII collagen (290 kd)
  - NC1 domain

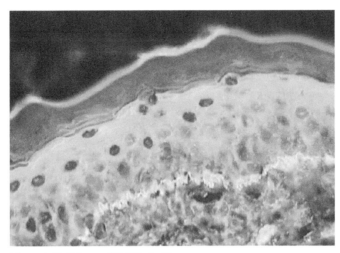

Fig.  1.7  Linear BMZ: IgG

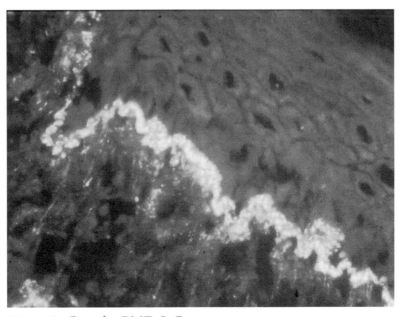

Fig.  1.8  Granular BMZ: IgG

# Epidermolysis Bullosa Acquisita

**Clinical**

- Erosions and blisters on trauma-prone areas such as elbows, knees, acral surfaces
- Scarring and milia, postinflammatory changes
- Nail dystrophy and scarring alopecia can occur
- Other variants: BP-like presentation, cicatricial pemphigoid-like presentation with mucous membrane involvement, Brunsting-Perry cicatricial pemphigoid-like presentation

**Direct Immunofluorescence**

- Linear BMZ: IgG (100%) and C3; occasionally IgA (66%) or IgM (50%)

**Indirect Immunofluorescence**

- Linear BMZ: IgG in 50% of patients
- SSS: dermal pattern (Fig. 1.9)

**Target Antigens**

- Type VII collagen (290 kd)
  - NC1 domain

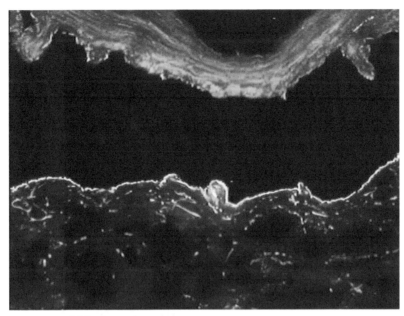

Fig. 1.9 SSS: dermal pattern

# Linear IgA Bullous Dermatosis

**Clinical**

- Widespread vesicles and bullae on normal skin or urticarial plaques
- Most commonly involves trunk
- Annular or targetoid appearance with peripheral vesicles or bullae
- Mucous membrane involvement is common, and ocular involvement also occurs
- Same disease as chronic bullous disease of childhood
- In chronic bullous disease of childhood: perineal and perioral involvement is very common
- Grouped small vesicles forming "clusters of jewels or pearls"

**Direct Immunofluorescence**

- Linear BMZ: IgA needed for diagnosis (less intense linear BMZ deposition of IgG, IgM, C3 in some cases) (Fig. 1.10)

**Indirect Immunofluorescence**

- Linear BMZ: IgA in 30% to 50% of cases (70% in chronic bullous disease of childhood)
- SSS: epidermal, dermal, or combined

**Target Antigens**

- BP180 (BPAG1)
- LABD (97 kd) and LAD-1 (120 kd) represent cleavage products of BP180
- Type VII collagen (290 kd) and a 285-kd dermal antigen

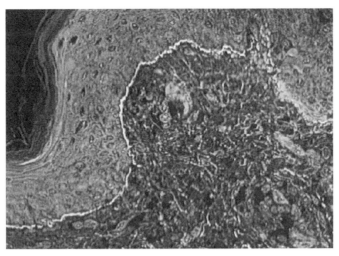

Fig. 1.10  Linear BMZ: IgA

# Cell Surface/Intercellular Space (ICS) Staining Pattern

A. Pemphigus Vulgaris

B. Pemphigus Vegetans

C. Pemphigus Foliaceus

D. Paraneoplastic Pemphigus

E. Pemphigus Erythematosus

F. IgA Pemphigus

# Pemphigus Vulgaris

**Clinical**

- Most common subtype of pemphigus
- Flaccid bullae rupture, leaving denuded areas
- Oral involvement is often the initial manifestation, in approximately 60% of patients
- Positive Nikolsky sign
- Skin manifestations involve scalp, chest, back, intertriginous areas

**Direct Immunofluorescence**

- Cell surface/ICS pattern for IgG (90%-100%) or C3 (Fig. 2.1)

**Indirect Immunofluorescence**

- Cell surface/ICS pattern for IgG in 90% of active cases (Fig. 2.2)

**Target Antigens**

- Desmoglein 3 (130 kd)
- Desmoglein 1 (160 kd)
- Anti-desmoglein 3 (in oral pemphigus vulgaris)
- Anti-desmogleins 3 and 1 (in mucocutaneous disease)
- Enzyme-linked immunosorbent assay for desmogleins 3 and 1 available and correlates with disease activity

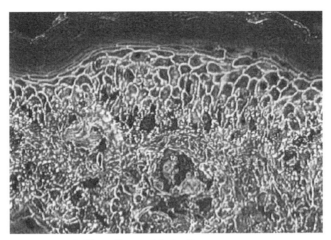

Fig.  2.1  Cell surface/ICS: IgG

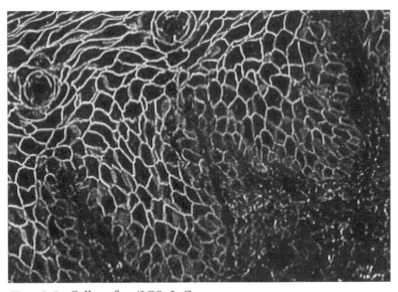

Fig.  2.2  Cell surface/ICS: IgG

# Pemphigus Vegetans

**Clinical**
- Variant of pemphigus vulgaris
- Painful flaccid bullae that lead to vegetative granulating lesions with or without pustules
- Involves intertriginous areas predominantly

**Direct Immunofluorescence**
- Identical to pemphigus vulgaris

**Indirect Immunofluorescence**
- Identical to pemphigus vulgaris

**Target Antigens**
- Identical to pemphigus vulgaris

# Pemphigus Foliaceus

**Clinical**

- Superficial vesicles or bullae that heal with superficial erosions and crusting
- Involves scalp, face, trunk
- No mucosal involvement
- Positive Nikolsky sign
- Pemphigus foliaceous variants:
  A. Fogo selvagem
  - Endemic in rural areas of Brazil
  - Correlates with blackfly (*Simulium* species) distribution
  - Increased familial tendency with increased HLA-DRB1
  B. Drug-induced pemphigus
  - More commonly associated with pemphigus foliaceus than pemphigus vulgaris (4:1)
  - Most common offending drugs: D-penicillamine, captopril

**Direct Immunofluorescence**

- Identical to pemphigus vulgaris (pg. 18)

**Indirect Immunofluorescence**

- Identical to pemphigus vulgaris (pg. 18)
- Guinea pig lip or esophagus also can be used (in addition to monkey esophagus)

**Target Antigens**

- Desmoglein 1 (160 kd)

# Paraneoplastic Pemphigus

**Clinical**
- Severe oral involvement
- Polymorphic cutaneous involvement
- Acral involvement occurs
- Associated bronchiolitis obliterans
- Associated malignancy
- In two-thirds of cases, tumor exists at presentation
- In one-third of cases, paraneoplastic pemphigus precedes the tumor

**Associated Neoplasms**
- Chronic lymphocytic leukemia
- Castleman tumor
- Thymoma
- Spindle cell neoplasms
- Waldenström macroglobulinemia

**Direct Immunofluorescence**
- Weak focal cell surface/ICS pattern and linear or granular BMZ for IgG or C3 (Fig. 2.3)
- Lichenoid changes also may be seen (shaggy BMZ and cytoid bodies)
- Increased rate of false-negative results

**Indirect Immunofluorescence**
- Cell surface/ICS (IgG) with or without linear BMZ on monkey esophagus substrate
- Rat bladder is most sensitive substrate for paraneoplastic pemphigus (Fig. 2.4)
  - 75% sensitive
  - 83% specific

**Target Antigens**
- Desmoglein 3 (130 kd)
- Desmoglein 1 (160 kd)
- Plectin (>500 kd)
- Desmoplakin I (250 kd)
- BP antigen I (230 kd)
- Desmoplakin II (210 kd)
- Envoplakin (210 kd)
- Periplakin (190 kd)
- 170 kd, undetermined

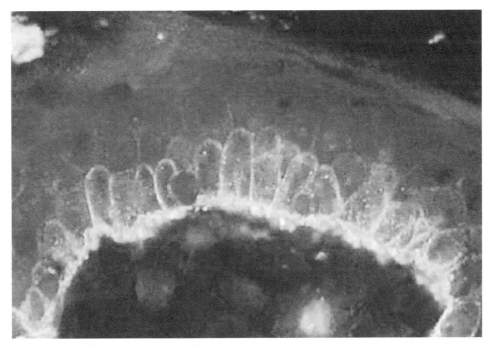

Fig. 2.3  Cell surface/ICS and linear BMZ: IgG

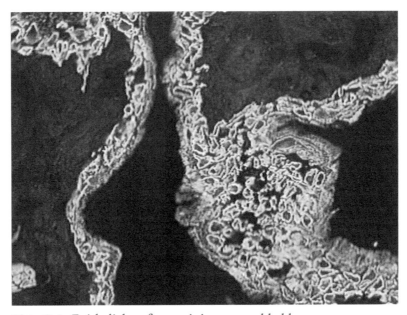

Fig. 2.4  Epithelial surface staining on rat bladder

# Pemphigus Erythematosus

| | |
|---|---|
| **Clinical** | ▪ Involves seborrheic areas of face and trunk, mimicking lupus erythematosus |
| **Direct Immunofluorescence** | ▪ Cell surface/ICS pattern (IgG or C3) and granular BMZ (IgM, C3) (Fig. 2.5 and 2.6) |
| **Indirect Immunofluorescence** | ▪ Cell surface/ICS pattern: IgG<br>▪ ANA |
| **Target Antigens** | ▪ Desmoglein 1 (160 kd) |

# IgA Pemphigus

| | |
|---|---|
| **Clinical** | ▪ Pruritic vesicles and pustules in an annular pattern<br>▪ Predilection for intertriginous areas<br>▪ Rare mucous membrane involvement<br>▪ Associated disorders<br>  - IgA monoclonal gammopathy<br>  - Crohn disease/gluten-sensitive enteropathy |
| **Direct Immunofluorescence** | ▪ Cell surface/ICS pattern for IgA  (Fig. 2.7) |
| **Indirect Immunofluorescence** | ▪ Positive in 50% of patients |
| **Target Antigens** | ▪ Desmocollin 1 (subset of patients target desmogleins 3 and 1) |

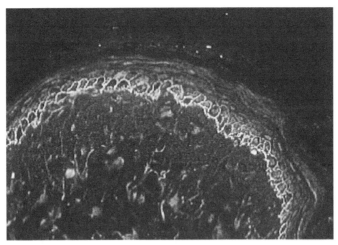

Fig. 2.5  Cell surface/ICS: IgG

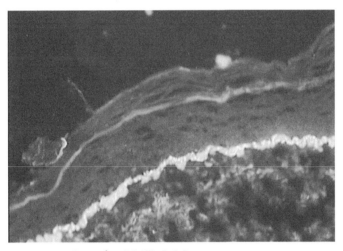

Fig. 2.6  Granular BMZ: IgM

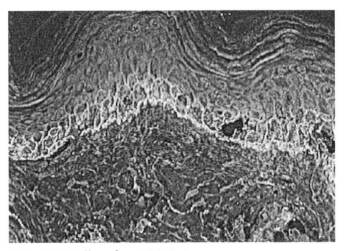

Fig. 2.7  Cell surface/ICS: IgA

# Granular Basement Membrane Zone Staining Pattern

A. Dermatitis Herpetiformis

B. Lupus Erythematosus

    1. Systemic Lupus Erythematosus

    2. Discoid Lupus Erythematosus

    3. Subacute Cutaneous Lupus Erythematosus

C. Mixed Connective Tissue Disease

D. Systemic Scleroderma

E. Dermatomyositis

# Dermatitis Herpetiformis

**Clinical**

- Erythematous papules or vesicles symmetrically distributed over extensor surfaces of the elbows, knees, buttocks, back, and scalp
- Vesicles may be grouped in a herpetiform configuration
- Intensely pruritic
- Often associated with multiple erosions caused by scratching
- One part of a spectrum of gluten-sensitive disorders that includes celiac disease
- An indirect consequence of a gluten-sensitive enteropathy

**Direct Immunofluorescence**

- Granular BMZ pattern for IgA, with stippling of dermal papillae (100%) (Fig. 3.1)
- Occasionally C3 (50%); IgG and IgM less often

**Indirect Immunofluorescence**

- IgA class endomysial antibody staining demonstrated in 76% of persons receiving a normal gluten-containing diet (Fig. 3.2)
- Endomysial antibody testing is recommended to identify a gluten-sensitive enteropathy and to monitor response to a gluten-free diet

**Target Antigens**

- Tissue transglutaminase in gluten-sensitive diseases
- Recent literature describing epidermal transglutaminase in skin lesions of dermatitis herpetiformis
- Circulating IgA antibody testing to tissue transglutaminase by enzyme-linked immunosorbent assay is recommended to identify the presence of a gluten-sensitive enteropathy and to monitor response to a gluten-free diet

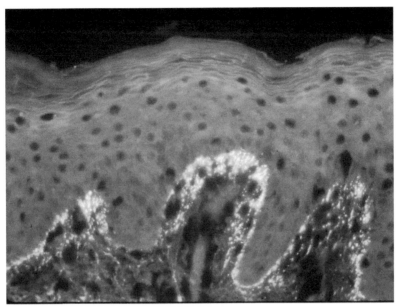

Fig. 3.1 Granular BMZ with stippling of dermal papillae: IgA

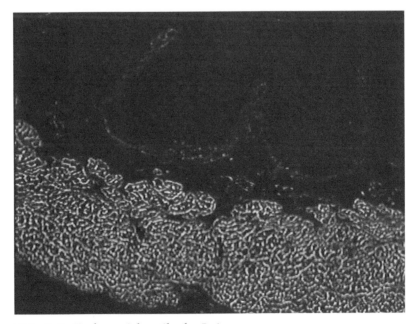

Fig. 3.2 Endomysial antibody: IgA

# Systemic Lupus Erythematosus

| | |
|---|---|
| **Clinical** | ▪ Malar "butterfly" rash |
| | ▪ Exacerbated by ultraviolet light |
| | ▪ Waxes and wanes with underlying systemic lupus erythematosus disease activity |
| | ▪ Discoid rash may occur at some point in the disease |
| | ▪ Photosensitivity |
| | ▪ Painless oral ulcers |
| | ▪ Nonerosive arthritis involving two or more peripheral joints |
| | ▪ Serositis |
| | ▪ Central nervous system involvement |
| | ▪ Nephritis |
| | ▪ Anemia, leukopenia, lymphopenia, thrombocytopenia |
| | ▪ See American College of Rheumatology's revised criteria for the classification of systemic lupus erythematosus (Tan et al, 1982) |
| | |
| **Immunologic Disorder** | ▪ ANA in abnormal titer |
| | ▪ Anti–double-stranded DNA in abnormal titer |
| | ▪ Presence of anti-Sm antibody |
| | ▪ IgG or IgM anticardiolipin antibodies |
| | |
| **Direct Immunofluorescence** | ▪ Granular BMZ pattern for IgG, IgM, IgA, C3 (Fig. 3.3) (sun-exposed involved skin >90%; sun-exposed nonlesional skin 50%; non–sun-exposed nonlesional skin 30%) |
| | ▪ Speckled epidermal nuclei pattern for IgG in 10% to 15% (Fig. 3.4) |
| | ▪ High yield with systemic lupus erythematosus–specific skin lesions: malar rash, erythematous edematous plaques, and active disease |
| | |
| **Indirect Immunofluorescence** | ▪ ANA |

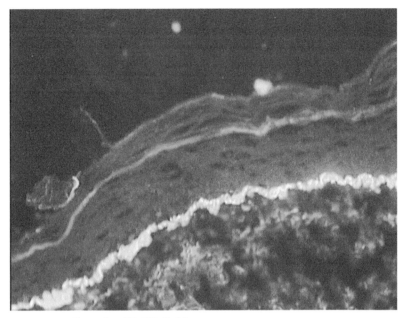

Fig. 3.3 Granular BMZ: IgM

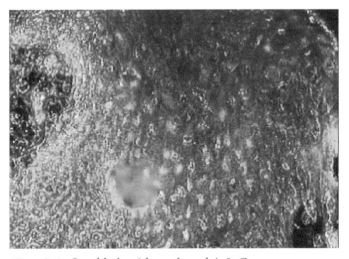

Fig. 3.4 Speckled epidermal nuclei: IgG

# Discoid Lupus Erythematosus

| | |
|---|---|
| **Clinical** | ▪ Discoid rash typically presents as sharply demarcated, erythematous, indurated plaques with hyperkeratosis, atrophy, telangiectasia, and follicular plugging |
| | ▪ Hypopigmentation or hyperpigmentation may be prominent |
| | ▪ Most frequently involves the face, scalp, ears, V area of the neck, and extensor aspects of the arms |
| | ▪ Scalp involvement may lead to scarring alopecia |
| **Immunologic Disorder** | ▪ Antibodies to single-stranded DNA may be present |
| | ▪ ANA present in low titers in 30% to 40% of patients |
| | ▪ Ro/SS-A and La/SS-B autoantibodies are rare |
| | ▪ Antibodies to double-stranded DNA are uncommon |
| **Direct Immunofluorescence** | ▪ Granular BMZ pattern for IgG and IgM (Fig. 3.5) (involved skin >90%) |
| | ▪ May have shaggy, thick BMZ with fibrinogen |
| | ▪ Cytoid bodies with IgM and IgA |
| **Indirect Immunofluorescence** | ▪ None (ANA rarely) |

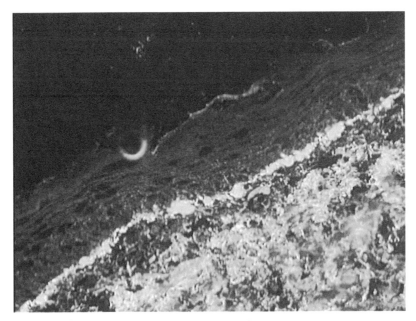

Fig. 3.5 Granular BMZ and cytoid bodies: IgM

# Subacute Cutaneous Lupus Erythematosus

**Clinical**
- Erythematous macules and papules that evolve into hyper-keratotic papulosquamous polycyclic and annular plaques
- Photosensitivity
- Less common on the face
- Heals without scarring
- May resolve with leukoderma and telangiectasias
- About 50% of patients meet the American College of Rheumatology's revised criteria for the classification of systemic lupus erythematosus

**Immunologic Disorder**
- Autoantibodies to Ro/SS-A ribonucleoprotein present in 70% to 90% strongly support the diagnosis
- Autoantibodies to La/SS-B present in 30% to 50%
- ANA present in 60% to 80%

**Direct Immunofluorescence**
- Granular BMZ pattern for IgG, IgM, C3
- Epidermal/keratinocyte intracytoplasmic particulate deposition with IgG (Fig. 3.6)
- Cytoid bodies for IgM and IgA

**Indirect Immunofluorescence**
- ANA

# Mixed Connective Tissue Disease

**Clinical**
- Combined features of lupus erythematosus, scleroderma, and myositis

**Immunologic Disorder**
- High titers of antibody to the extractable nuclear antigen

**Direct Immunofluorescence**
- Granular BMZ pattern rare (15%)
- Speckled epidermal nuclei for IgG in 46% to 100%

**Indirect Immunofluorescence**
- ANA

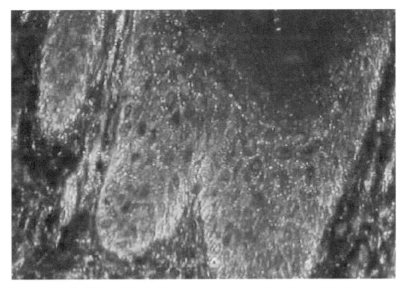

Fig. 3.6 Epidermal/keratinocyte intracytoplasmic particulate
deposition: IgG

# Systemic Scleroderma

**Clinical**

- Skin tightening extends from fingers to upper extremities, trunk, face, and, finally, lower extremities
- Raynaud phenomenon
- Nail-fold capillary changes (giant or sausage-shaped loops)
- Edema of the hands and fingers
- Flexion contractures and sclerodactyly with waxy, shiny, atrophic skin
- Ulcers on fingertips and over knuckles
- Masklike, expressionless face, with loss of normal facial lines
- Small, sharp nose, thinning of lips and hair
- Microstomia with radial furrowing around the mouth
- Matlike telangiestasias on face and upper trunk
- Esophageal dysfunction in more than 90%
- Pulmonary fibrosis
- Myocardial fibrosis in 50% to 70%
- Renal involvement with hypertension

**Immunologic Disorder**

- Anticentromere antibodies only in 12% to 25% of patients (present in 50%-96% of patients with CREST syndrome)
- Scl-70 autoantibodies (30%)

**Direct Immunofluorescence**

- Granular BMZ pattern for IgM (sun-exposed 60%)
- Speckled epidermal nuclei pattern in 20%
- Shaggy BMZ with fibrinogen (Fig. 3.7)

**Indirect Immunofluorescence**

- ANA

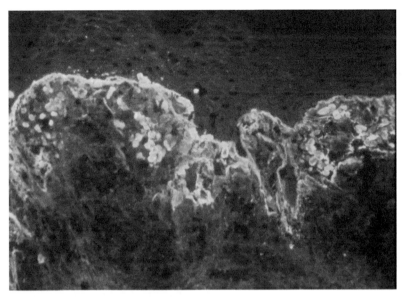

Fig. 3.7  Shaggy BMZ: fibrinogen

# Dermatomyositis

**Clinical**

- Erythematous, violaceous papules over the dorsal aspect of the interphalangeal or metacarpophalangeal joints (termed Gottron papules)
- Symmetric, confluent, violaceous erythema over the interphalangeal or metacarpophalangeal joints, olecranon process, medial malleoli, and patella (termed Gottron sign)
- Periorbital, violaceous (heliotrope) erythema and edema
- Periungual telangiectasia with or without cuticular hemorrhage and dystrophic cuticles
- Violaceous erythema over dorsal aspect of arms, posterior aspect of shoulder and neck (shawl sign)
- Poikiloderma atrophicans
- Pruritus can be severe
- Cutaneous calcification is more common in juvenile form (40%-50%)
- Symmetric proximal muscle weakness
- Skeletal muscle-derived enzymes increased in 90% of cases of classic dermatomyositis at some point of the disease
- Abnormal muscle biopsy specimen
- Abnormal electromyographic results
- Higher-than-expected risk for malignancy (ovarian cancer), especially in patients 50 years or older

**Immunologic Disorder**

- Increased ANA levels on human tumor cell substrates (60%-80%)
- Anti-Jo-1 (20% of cases of classic dermatomyositis and 40% of cases of polymyositis)

**Direct Immunofluorescence**

- Granular BMZ pattern for IgM, IgG, and C3 (low intensity)
- Cytoid bodies for IgM (Fig. 3.8) and IgA, shaggy BMZ with fibrinogen (Fig. 3.9)

**Indirect Immunofluorescence**

- ANA

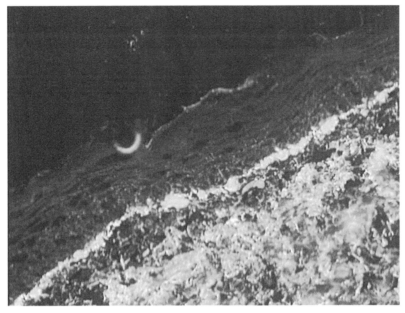

Fig. 3.8 Granular BMZ and cytoid bodies: IgM

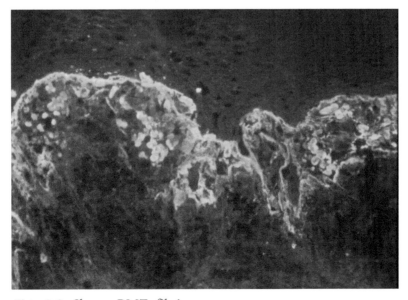

Fig. 3.9 Shaggy BMZ: fibrinogen

# Shaggy Basement Membrane Zone Staining Pattern

# Lichenoid Tissue Reactions

**Clinical**

Lichen planus

- Erythematous to violaceous, flat-topped, polygonal papules with fine, whitish reticulations termed Wickham striae
- Distributed symmetrically over flexural areas of extremities
- Pruritus usually present
- Hypertrophic lichen planus extremely pruritic
- Presence of Koebner phenomenon
- White, reticulated pattern occurs with oral involvement
- Nail pterygium or complete loss of nail plate

Lupus erythematosus and other connective tissue disorders

- See Chapter III

Lichenoid drug reactions

- Initiated by many drugs, such as β-adrenergic blockers (latent period of 1 year), penicillamine (latent period of 2 months-3 years), angiotensin-converting enzyme inhibitors, especially captopril (latent period of 3-6 months)
- Usually resolves 2 to 4 months after discontinuation of offending drug

Lichenoid photodermatoses

- Lesions appear eczematous with a photodistributed pattern
- Drugs that induce a photodistributed lichenoid reaction include carbamazepine, chlorpromazine, ethambutol, quinine, tetracyclines, thiazide diuretics, and furosemide
- Generally resolve 3 to 4 months from discontinuation of offending drug

**Direct Immunofluorescence**

- Shaggy BMZ pattern for fibrinogen (Fig. 4.1)
- Cytoid bodies for IgM and IgA, occasionally IgG, C3, and fibrinogen (Fig. 4.2)

**Indirect Immunofluorescence**

- ANA for lupus erythematosus

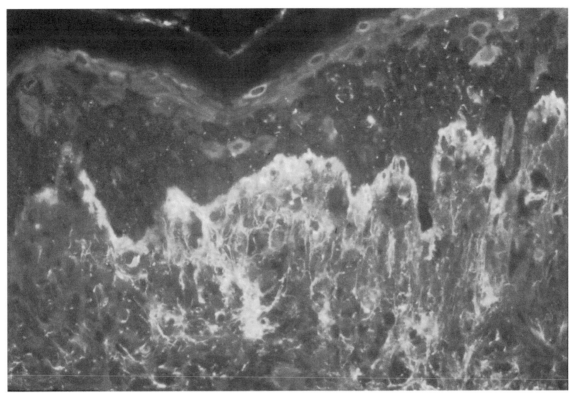

**Fig. 4.1** Shaggy BMZ: fibrinogen

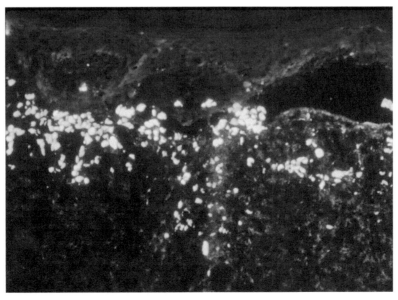

**Fig. 4.2** Scattered and clumped cytoid bodies: IgM

# Vascular Staining Pattern and Others

A. Porphyria

B. Henoch-Schönlein Purpura

C. Vasculitis

# Porphyria

**Clinical**

Porphyria cutanea tarda

- Most common porphyria
- Photosensitivity, fragile skin
- Vesicles, bullae, erosions, crusts, milia, scarring, hypertrichosis on sun-exposed areas
- Usually occurs in third or fourth decade of life
- Most often acquired, but autosomal dominant in 20% of cases
- Associated with use of oral contraceptives, alcohol, chemicals (hexachlorobenzene, chlorinated phenols)

Pseudoporphyria

- Clinically identical to porphyria cutanea tarda
- Associated with chronic renal failure with hemodialysis, systemic lupus erythematosus, hepatoma, hepatitis C, sarcoidosis, drugs
- Offending drugs include nonsteroidal anti-inflammatory drugs, tetracyclines, nalidixic acid, furosemide, diazide, cyclosporine

**Direct Immunofluorescence**

- Dermal vessels: homogeneous thick staining pattern for IgG, ± IgA, C3, fibrinogen (Fig. 5.1)
- Granular BMZ for C3, IgM
- Weak, thick linear BMZ for IgG, IgA

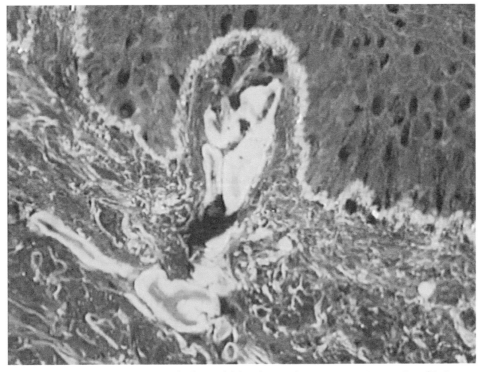

**Fig. 5.1** Homogeneous thick dermal blood vessels: IgG, IgA, IgM, C3, fibrinogen

# Henoch-Schönlein Purpura

Clinical
- Predominantly occurs in children but can occur in adults
- Palpable purpura over the feet, ankles, lower extremities
- Recent upper respiratory tract infection in 75% of cases
- Abdominal pain, gastrointestinal bleeding, or intussusception
- Arthralgia, arthritis
- Glomerulonephritis

Direct Immunofluorescence
- Strong dermal vessels with IgA (± other conjugates) (Fig. 5.2)

# Vasculitis

Clinical
- Palpable purpura
- Macules, urticaria, pustules, vesicles, ulcers, necrosis, and livedo reticularis may be present
- Most often involves lower extremities or other dependent areas
- Specific diagnosis is dependent on the organ pattern involvement and histopathologic findings

Direct Immunofluorescence
- Strong dermal vessels with IgM, IgG, C3, fibrinogen (Fig. 5.3)

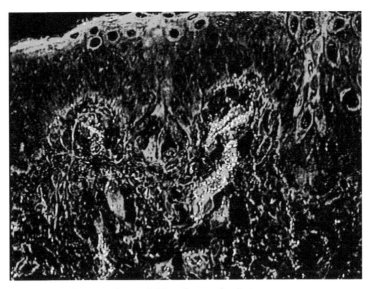

Fig. 5.2 Strong dermal blood vessels: IgA

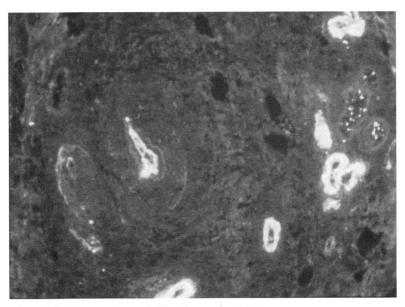

Fig. 5.3 Strong dermal blood vessels: IgM

# Summary

## Summary Table

| Disease | Direct immunofluorescence | Indirect immunofluorescence | Target antigens |
|---|---|---|---|
| | Linear BMZ staining pattern | | |
| **Bullous pemphigoid** | Linear BMZ: IgG (90%) and C3 (>90%, nearly all)<br><br><br>*Linear BMZ (IgG)* | BMZ antibodies (IgG) in 75%<br><br>SSS: epidermal pattern (shown below), occasionally combined epidermal-dermal pattern<br><br><br>*BMZ antibodies (IgG)*<br><br><br>*Epidermal pattern (IgG)* | BP230<br><br>BP180<br>▪ NC16A |
| **Pemphigoid gestationis (herpes gestationis)** | Linear BMZ: C3 (100%); IgG (approximately 25%) | BMZ antibodies (IgG) in <25%<br><br>HG factor in 50%<br><br>SSS: epidermal pattern | BP230<br><br>BP180<br>▪ NC16A |

## Lichen planus pemphigoides

Linear BMZ: IgG and C3 with changes of lichen planus (cytoid bodies with IgM, IgA, C3, and shaggy BMZ with fibrinogen)

BMZ antibodies (IgG) in 50%

SSS: epidermal pattern

BP230

BP180

■ NC16A

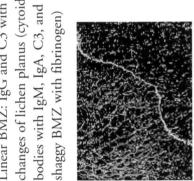

*Linear BMZ (IgG)*

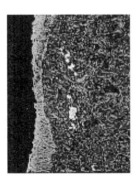

*Cytoid bodies (IgA)*

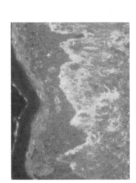

*Shaggy BMZ (fibrinogen)*

| Disease | Direct immunofluorescence | Indirect immunofluorescence | Target antigens |
| --- | --- | --- | --- |
| | | Linear BMZ staining pattern | |
| **Mucous membrane pemphigoid** | Linear BMZ: IgG, C3, or IgA | BMZ antibodies (IgG) in 15%–20%<br><br>SSS: epidermal, dermal, or combined<br><br><br>*Dermal pattern (IgG)* | BP230<br><br>BP180<br>■ C-terminus and some NC16A<br><br>$\beta_4$ integrin subunit<br><br>Laminin-5 (also called epiligrin, nicein, kalinin, BM600)<br><br>Laminin-6<br><br>Type VII collagen (290 kd) |
| **Bullous lupus erythematosus** | Linear BMZ: IgG and C3; IgM and IgA also | ANA<br><br>BMZ antibodies not detected on monkey esophagus can be detected on SSS (dermal pattern) | Type VII collagen (290 kd)<br>■ NC1 domain |
| **Epidermolysis bullosa acquisita** | Linear BMZ: IgG (100%) and C3; occasionally IgA (66%) or IgM (50%) | BMZ antibodies (IgG) in 50%<br><br>SSS: dermal pattern | Type VII collagen (290 kd)<br>■ NC1 domain |

**Linear IgA bullous dermatosis**

Linear BMZ: IgA needed for diagnosis; less intense deposition of IgG, IgM, and C3 in some cases

*Linear BMZ (IgA)*

BMZ antibodies (IgA) in 30%-50% (70% in chronic bullous disease of childhood)

SSS: epidermal, dermal, or combined

*Dermal pattern (IgA)*

BP180

LABD (97 kd) and LAD-1 (120 kd) represent cleavage products of BP180

Type VII collagen (290 kd) and a 285-kd dermal antigen

## Cell surface/ICS staining pattern

**Pemphigus vulgaris and vegetans**

ICS: IgG (90%-100%) or C3

*ICS (IgG)*

ICS antibodies (IgG) in 90% of active cases

*ICS (IgG)*

Desmoglein 3 (130 kd)

Desmoglein 1 (160 kd)

**Pemphigus foliaceus**

ICS: IgG (90%-100%) or C3

ICS antibodies (IgG)

Guinea pig lip or esophagus: ICS antibodies (IgG)

Desmoglein 1 (160 kd)

| Disease | Direct immunofluorescence | Indirect immunofluorescence | Target antigens |
|---|---|---|---|
| | | Cell surface/ICS staining pattern | |
| **Paraneoplastic pemphigus** | ICS: IgG (90%-100%) and C3 | ICS antibodies (IgG); BMZ antibodies (IgG) | Desmoglein 1 (160 kd) |
| | BMZ: linear or granular (C3, IgG) | Rat bladder epithelium (best screening: 83% specific, 75% sensitive). ICS antibodies, occasionally BMZ | Desmoglein 3 (130 kd) |
| | | | Plectin (>500 kd) |
| | May have lichenoid changes (cytoid bodies with IgM and IgA, rarely C3 and shaggy BMZ with fibrinogen) | | Desmoplakin I (250 kd) |
| | | | BP antigen I (230kd) |
| | | | Desmoplakin II (210 kd) |
| | | | Envoplakin (210 kd) |
| | | | Periplakin (190 kd) |
| | | | 170 kd, undetermined |

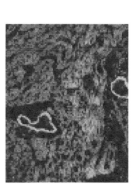

*Rat bladder (IgG)*

*Mouse liver, portal ducts (IgG)*

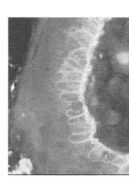

*ICS and linear BMZ (IgG)*

## Pemphigus erythematosus

Desmoglein 1 (160 kd)

ICS antibodies (IgG)

ANA

ICS: IgG or C3

BMZ: granular IgM, C3

*ICS (IgG)*

*Granular BMZ (IgM)*

## IgA pemphigus

Desmocollin 1 (subset of patients target desmogleins 3 and 1)

ICS antibodies (IgA) in 50%

ICS: IgA

*ICS (IgA)*

| Disease | Direct immunofluorescence | Indirect immunofluorescence | Target antigens |
|---|---|---|---|
| | | Granular BMZ staining pattern | |
| **Dermatitis herpetiformis** | Granular BMZ: IgA, with stippling of dermal papillae (100%); occasionally C3 (50%), IgG and IgM less often<br><br>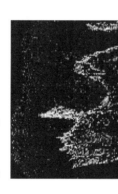<br>*Granular BMZ with stippling of dermal papillae (IgA)* | IgA class endomysial antibodies in 76% of those on a normal gluten-containing diet<br><br>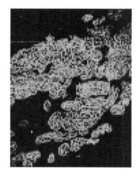<br>*Endomysial antibody (IgA)* | Tissue transglutaminase in gluten-sensitive diseases<br><br>Recent literature describing epidermal transglutaminase in skin lesions of dermatitis herpetiformis<br><br>Circulating IgA antibody testing to tissue transglutaminase by enzyme-linked immunosorbent assay is recommended to identify the presence of a gluten-sensitive enteropathy and to monitor response to a gluten-free diet |

**Lupus erythematosus**

**Systemic lupus erythematosus**

ANA

Granular BMZ: IgG, IgM, IgA, C3 (sun-exposed involved skin >90%; sun-exposed nonlesional skin 50%; non–sun-exposed nonlesional skin 30%)

Epidermal nuclei, speckled (IgG) in 10%–15%

High yield with systemic lupus erythematosus–specific skin lesions: malar rash, erythematous edematous plaques, and active disease

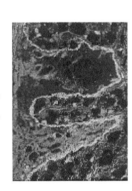

*Granular BMZ (IgM)*

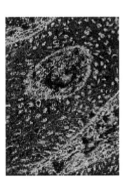

*Epidermal nuclei (IgG)*

| Disease | Direct immunofluorescence | Indirect immunofluorescence | Target antigens |
|---|---|---|---|
| | Granular BMZ staining pattern | | |
| **Discoid lupus erythematosus** | Granular BMZ: IgG and IgM (involved skin >90%)<br><br>May have shaggy thick bands<br><br>Cytoid bodies with IgM and IgA | None (ANA rarely) | |

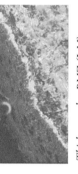

*Thick granular BMZ (IgM)*

**Subacute cutaneous lupus erythematosus**

Granular BMZ: IgG, IgM, C3    ANA

Epidermal/keratinocyte intracytoplasmic particulate deposition (IgG)

Cytoid bodies (IgM and IgA)

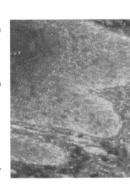

*Intracytoplasmic particulate deposition (IgG)*

**Mixed connective tissue disease**

Granular BMZ: rare (15%)    ANA

Epidermal nuclei, speckled (IgG) in 46%–100%

**Systemic scleroderma**

Granular BMZ: IgM (sun-exposed 60%)    ANA

Epidermal nuclei, speckled, in 20%

**Dermatomyositis**

Granular BMZ: IgM, IgG, and C3 (low intensity)    ANA

Cytoid bodies, IgM and IgA

| Disease | Direct immunofluorescence | Indirect immunofluorescence | Target antigens |
|---|---|---|---|
| | | Shaggy BMZ staining pattern | |
| **Lichenoid tissue reactions** | | | |
| **Lichen planus** | Shaggy BMZ: fibrinogen | None | |
| **Lupus erythematosus** | Cytoid bodies (IgM and IgA, occasionally IgG, C3, and fibrinogen) | ANA for systemic lupus erythematosus | |
| **Drug reactions** | | | |
| **Photodermatoses** | | | |

*Cytoid bodies (IgM)*

*Shaggy BMZ (fibrinogen)*

## Vascular staining pattern and others

**Porphyria**

Dermal vessels: homogeneous IgG, granular C3

None

BMZ: weak, thick linear BMZ

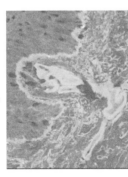

*Homogeneous thick dermal blood vessels: IgG, IgA, IgM, C3, fibrinogen*

**Henoch-Schönlein purpura**

Strong dermal vessels: IgA

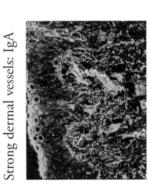

*Dermal vessels (IgA)*

| Disease | Direct immunofluorescence | Indirect immunofluorescence | Target antigens |
|---|---|---|---|
| | Vascular staining pattern and others | | |
| Vasculitis | Strong dermal vessels: IgM ± C3, IgG *Dermal vessels (IgM)* *Dermal vessels (C3)* | | |

# Immunofluorescence Flowchart

1. **Linear BMZ (DIF)**
   ▓ **Linear BMZ: IgG, C3 ± IgA**
   • IIF on SSS
      – Epidermal pattern:
         i. Bullous pemphigoid and its variants
         ii. Mucous membrane pemphigoid
         iii. Lichen planus pemphigoides
      – Dermal pattern:
         i. Bullous systemic lupus erythematosus
         ii. Epidermolysis bullosa acquisita
         iii. Mucous membrane pemphigoid
         iv. Brunsting-Perry cicatricial pemphigoid
   ▓ **Linear BMZ: IgG, C3**
      + lichenoid changes (cytoid bodies with IgM and IgA and shaggy BMZ with fibrinogen)
         i. Lichen planus pemphigoides
   ▓ **Linear BMZ: IgA ± IgG, C3**
      • IIF with IgA may show an epidermal, dermal, or combined pattern
         i. Linear IgA bullous disease or chronic bullous disease of childhood
   ▓ **Linear BMZ: C3 ± IgG**
      • HG factor:
         i. Pemphigoid (herpes) gestationis

2. **ICS/cell surface (DIF)**
   ▓ **ICS: IgG, C3**
      • IIF with monkey esophagus
         – Positive:
            i. Pemphigus vulgaris
            ii. Pemphigus vegetans
            iii. Pemphigus foliaceus
      • IIF with guinea pig esophagus/lip
         i. Pemphigus foliaceus
   ▓ **ICS: IgG, C3**
      + linear/granular BMZ (C3, IgG) + lichenoid changes (cytoid bodies with IgM and IgA and shaggy BMZ with fibrinogen)
         i. Paraneoplastic pemphigus
   ▓ **ICS: IgG, C3**
      + granular BMZ (IgM ± other conjugates) ± ANA
         i. Pemphigus erythematosus
   ▓ **ICS: IgA**
         i. IgA pemphigus

3. **Granular BMZ (DIF)**
   ▓ **Granular BMZ: IgA, with stippling of the dermal papillae**
         i. Dermatitis herpetiformis (confirm with tissue transglutaminase ELISA or IIF with endomysial antibody)
   ▓ **Granular BMZ: IgG, IgM, C3**
      ± epidermal nuclear fluorescence (speckled) ± lichenoid tissue reaction ± epidermal intracyto-plasmic particulate deposition
         i. Lupus erythematosus

4. **Shaggy BMZ (DIF)**
   ▓ **Shaggy BMZ: fibrinogen**
      + cytoid bodies (IgA, IgM)
      • Lichenoid tissue reactions
         i. Lichen planus
         ii. Lichenoid drug reactions
         iii. Connective tissue diseases
   ▓ **Shaggy BMZ: fibrinogen (mucosa)**
         i. Lichenoid tissue reaction
         ii. Oral lichen planus
         iii. Lichenoid drug reactions
         iv. Oral lupus erythematosus

5. **Epidermal nuclear fluorescence (anti-U1RNP) (DIF)**
         i. Mixed connective tissue disease (47%-100%)
         ii. Systemic scleroderma (20%)
         iii. Systemic lupus erythematosus (10%-15%)

6. **Epidermal/keratinocyte intracytoplasmic particulate staining with IgG (anti-Ro/SS-A) (DIF)**
         i. Subacute cutaneous lupus erythematosus
         ii. Sjögren syndrome
         iii. Mixed connective tissue disease

7. **Thickened BMZ and dermal vessels (DIF)**
   ▓ **Thickened linear BMZ: IgG**
      + homogeneous vessels (IgG) and granular vessels (C3)
         i. Porphyria

8. **Strong dermal vessels (DIF)**
   ▓ **Dermal blood vessels: IgG or IgM or IgA or C3 (2 or more conjugates required)**
         i. Vasculitis
   ▓ **Dermal blood vessels: IgA**
         i. Henoch-Schönlein purpura

DIF, direct immunofluorescence; ELISA, enzyme-linked immunosorbent assay; IIF, indirect immunofluorescence.

# Practice Questions for Board Exams

1. **A 55-year-old man presents with multiple flaccid bullae on his trunk which are short-lived and develop crusts. He does not have mucosal involvement. The patient most likely has:**

   a. Bullous pemphigoid
   b. Cicatricial pemphigoid
   c. Pemphigus vulgaris
   d. Pemphigus foliaceus
   e. Dermatitis herpetiformis

2. **The following immunofluorescence pattern is with fluorescein-labeled IgA. The patient's diagnosis is:**

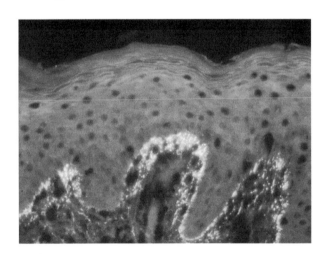

   a. Linear IgA bullous dermatitis
   b. Dermatitis herpetiformis
   c. IgA pemphigus
   d. Cicatricial pemphigoid
   e. Lupus erythematosus

3. **The following indirect immunofluorescence pattern on SSS can be found in:**

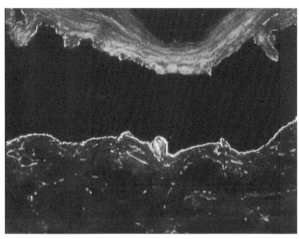

   a. Pemphigus vulgaris
   b. Pemphigus foliaceus
   c. Bullous pemphigoid
   d. Pemphigoid gestationis
   e. Epidermolysis bullosa acquisita

4. **In a 30-year-old woman, a vesicular eruption develops on her trunk 2 days post partum. The most specific diagnostic pattern on direct immunofluorescence is:**

   a. Strong granular BMZ with IgG
   b. Cell surface/ICS pattern with C3
   c. Strong linear BMZ with C3
   d. Shaggy BMZ staining with fibrinogen
   e. Cytoid bodies with IgM

5. **The following immunofluorescence pattern is seen with IgG. The most likely diagnosis is:**

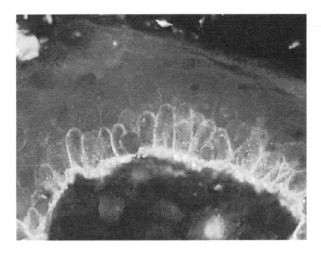

   a. Bullous pemphigoid
   b. Mucous membrane pemphigoid
   c. Pemphigus foliaceus
   d. Paraneoplastic pemphigus
   e. Pemphigus vulgaris

6. **A patient has only positive desmoglein-1 antibodies. The patient has:**

   a. Pemphigus vulgaris
   b. Pemphigus foliaceus
   c. Paraneoplastic pemphigus
   d. IgA pemphigus
   e. Bullous pemphigoid

7. **The following immunofluorescence pattern is seen with IgA. The patient has:**

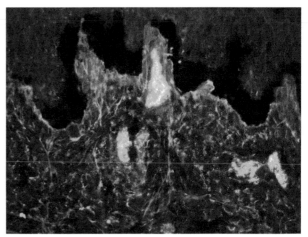

   a. Dermatitis herpetiformis
   b. Linear IgA bullous dermatitis
   c. IgA pemphigus
   d. Henoch-Schönlein purpura
   e. Porphyria

8. **A 45-year-old woman presents with photosensitivity and bullae. She has autoantibodies directed against:**

   a. BP180
   b. Desmoglein 3
   c. Desmoglein 1
   d. Desmogleins 3 and 1
   e. Type VII collagen

9. **The following immunofluorescence pattern is seen with IgM. The patient most likely has:**

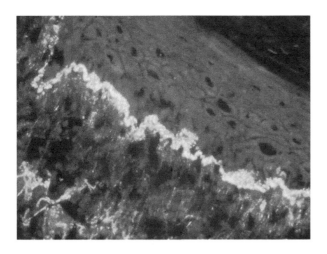

   a. Bullous pemphigoid
   b. Lupus erythematosus
   c. Cicatricial pemphigoid
   d. Epidermolysis bullosa acquisita
   e. Dermatitis herpetiformis

10. **The following immunofluorescence pattern is seen with IgA. The patient's autoantibodies are most likely to react against:**

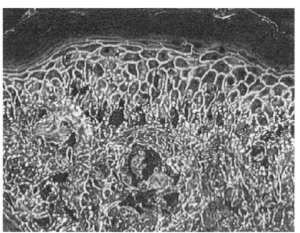

   a. Desmoglein 3
   b. Desmoglein 1
   c. Desmocollin 1
   d. Desmogleins 3 and 1
   e. Periplakin

11. **A 59-year-old woman has a linear dermal pattern with IgG on SSS and an associated malignancy. The diagnosis is most likely:**

   a. Paraneoplastic pemphigus
   b. Antiepiligrin cicatricial pemphigoid
   c. Bullous pemphigoid
   d. Celiac disease
   e. Epidermolysis bullosa acquisita

12. **The following direct immunofluorescence photograph shows staining with fibrinogen. The most likely diagnosis is:**

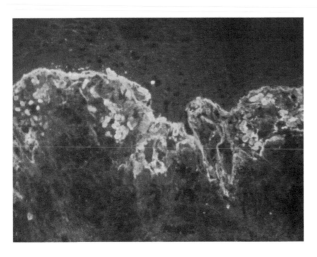

a. Bullous pemphigoid
b. Pemphigus vulgaris
c. Systemic lupus erythematosus
d. Epidermolysis bullosa acquisita
e. Lichen planus

13. **The most sensitive substrate for the diagnosis of paraneoplastic pemphigus by immunofluorescence is:**

a. Rat bladder
b. Monkey esophagus
c. Guinea pig esophagus
d. SSS
e. Guinea pig lip

14. **An 80-year-old patient presents with multiple tense bullae. The most important autoantibodies are targeting:**

a. BP230
b. BP180
c. NC16A domain of BP180
d. NC1 domain of type VII collagen
e. Desmogleins 3 and 1

15. **The following immunofluorescence pattern is seen with IgG. The most likely diagnosis is:**

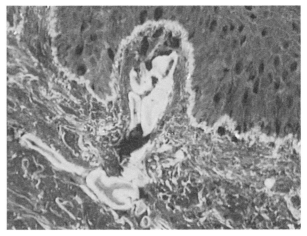

a. Leukocytoclastic vasculitis
b. Henoch-Schönlein purpura
c. Bullous pemphigoid
d. Porphyria
e. Epidermolysis bullosa acquisita

16. **The target antigen in antiepiligrin cicatricial pemphigoid is:**

    a. Desmoglein 3
    b. Desmoglein 1
    c. Desmogleins 3 and 1
    d. Laminin 5
    e. Type VII collagen

17. **A 45-year-old patient presents with an annular skin eruption characterized by peripheral vesicles. The characteristic immunofluorescence pattern seen on a direct immunofluorescence biopsy is:**

    a. Linear BMZ staining for IgG
    b. Cell surface staining for C3
    c. Linear BMZ staining for IgA
    d. Linear BMZ staining for C3
    e. Granular BMZ staining for IgM

18. **The following staining pattern for IgG on direct immunofluorescence is most commonly seen in:**

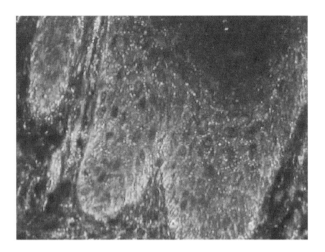

    a. Subacute cutaneous lupus erythematosus
    b. Epidermolysis bullosa acquisita
    c. Discoid lupus erythematosus
    d. Pemphigoid gestationis
    e. Cicatricial pemphigoid

19. **The following staining pattern seen for IgA is characteristic of:**

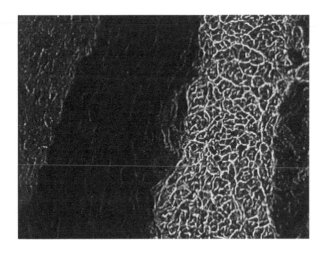

a. Pemphigus vulgaris
b. Celiac disease
c. Pemphigus foliaceus
d. Paraneoplastic pemphigus
e. Bullous pemphigoid


20. **The following is a target antigen recognized in paraneoplastic pemphigus:**

a. BP230
b. Type VII collagen
c. NC16A domain of BP180
d. Desmocollin 1
e. Periplakin

# Answers

| | | | |
|---|---|---|---|
| 1. | d | 11. | b |
| 2. | b | 12. | e |
| 3. | e | 13. | a |
| 4. | c | 14. | c |
| 5. | d | 15. | d |
| 6. | b | 16. | d |
| 7. | d | 17. | c |
| 8. | e | 18. | a |
| 9. | b | 19. | b |
| 10. | c | 20. | e |

# Suggested Reading

Anhalt GJ, Kim SC, Stanley JR, Korman NJ, Jabs DA, Kory M, et al. Paraneoplastic pemphigus: an autoimmune mucocutaneous disease associated with neoplasia. N Engl J Med. 1990;323:1729-35.

Beutner EN, Jordon RE. Demonstration of skin antibodies in sera of pemphigus vulgaris patients by indirect immunofluorescent staining. Proc Soc Exp Biol Med. 1964;117:505-10.

Brunsting LA, Perry HO. Benign pemphigoid; a report of seven cases with chronic, scarring, herpetiform plaques about the head and neck. AMA Arch Derm. 1957;75:489-501.

Caproni M, Cardinali C, Renzi D, Calabro A, Fabbri P. Tissue transglutaminase antibody assessment in dermatitis herpetiformis. Br J Dermatol. 2001;144:196-7.

Chan LS. Mucous membrane pemphigoid. Clin Dermatol. 2001;19:703-11.

Chan LS, Ahmed AR, Anhalt GJ, Bernauer W, Cooper KD, Elder MJ, et al. The first international consensus on mucous membrane pemphigoid: definition, diagnostic criteria, pathogenic factors, medical treatment, and prognostic indicators. Arch Dermatol. 2002;138:370-9.

Dahl MV. Clinical immunodermatology. 3rd ed. St. Louis: Mosby; 1996.

Diaz LA, Giudice GJ. End of the century overview of skin blisters. Arch Dermatol. 2000;136:106-12.

Ghohestani RF, Li K, Rousselle P, Uitto J. Molecular organization of the cutaneous basement membrane zone. Clin Dermatol. 2001;19:551-62.

Guide SV, Marinkovich MP. Linear IgA bullous dermatosis. Clin Dermatol. 2001;19:719-27.

Hall RP III. Dermatitis herpetiformis. J Invest Dermatol. 1992;99:873-81.

Hallel-Halevy D, Nadelman C, Chen M, Woodley DT. Epidermolysis bullosa acquisita: update and review. Clin Dermatol. 2001;19:712-8.

Hashimoto T. Immunopathology of IgA pemphigus. Clin Dermatol. 2001;19:683-9.

Hashimoto T. Immunopathology of paraneoplastic pemphigus. Clin Dermatol. 2001;19:675-82.

Ishii K, Amagai M, Komai A, Ebihara T, Chorzelski TP, Jablonska S, et al. Desmoglein 1 and desmoglein 3 are the target autoantigens in herpetiform pemphigus. Arch Dermatol. 1999;135:943-7.

Jenkins RE, Shornick JK, Black MM. Pemphigoid gestationis. J Eur Acad Dermatol Venereol. 1993;2:163-73.

Jordon RE. Atlas of bullous disease. New York: Churchill Livingstone; 2000

Jordon RE, Schroeter AL, Rogers RS III, Perry HO. Classical and alternate pathway activation of complement in pemphigus vulgaris lesions. J Invest Dermatol. 1974;63:256-9.

Kalaaji AN, Rogers RS III, Stone RM. Pemphigoid nodularis. Int J Immunopathol Pharmacol. (in press).

Korman NJ. Bullous pemphigoid. Dermatol Clin. 1993;11:483-98.

Lin MS, Arteaga LA, Diaz LA. Herpes gestationis. Clin Dermatol. 2001;19:697-702.

Martel P, Joly P. Pemphigus: autoimmune diseases of keratinocyte's adhesion molecules. Clin Dermatol. 2001;19:662-74.

Mutasim DF, Adams BB. Immunofluorescence in dermatology. J Am Acad Dermatol. 2001;45:803-22.

Nguyen VT, Ndoye A, Bassler KD, Shultz LD, Shields MC, Ruben BS, et al. Classification, clinical manifestations, and immunopathological mechanisms of the epithelial variant of paraneoplastic autoimmune multiorgan syndrome: a reappraisal of paraneoplastic pemphigus. Arch Dermatol. 2001;137:193-206.

Nguyen VT, Ndoye A, Grando SA. Pemphigus vulgaris antibody identifies pemphaxin: a novel keratinocyte annexin-like molecule binding acetylcholine. J Biol Chem. 2000;275:29466-76.

Nicolas ME, Krause PK, Gibson LE, Murray JA. Dermatitis herpetiformis. Int J Dermatol. 2003;42:588-600.

Nishikawa T, Hashimoto T. Dermatoses with intraepidermal IgA deposits. Clin Dermatol. 2000;18:315-8.

Pas HH. Immunoblot assay in differential diagnosis of autoimmune blistering skin diseases. Clin Dermatol. 2001;19:622-30.

Porter WM, Unsworth DJ, Lock RJ, Hardman CM, Baker BS, Fry L. Tissue transglutaminase antibodies in dermatitis herpetiformis. Gastroenterology. 1999;117:749-50.

Proby C, Fujii Y, Owaribe K, Nishikawa T, Amagai M. Human autoantibodies against HD1/plectin in paraneoplastic pemphigus. J Invest Dermatol. 1999;112:153-6.

Reunala TL. Dermatitis herpetiformis. Clin Dermatol. 2001;19:728-36.

Robinson ND, Hashimoto T, Amagai M, Chan LS. The new pemphigus variants. J Am Acad Dermatol. 1999;40:649-71.

Rogers RS III, Seehafer JR, Perry HO. Treatment of cicatricial (benign mucous membrane) pemphigoid with dapsone. J Am Acad Dermatol. 1982;6:215-23.

Rose C, Dieterich W, Brocker EB, Schuppan D, Zillikens D. Circulating autoantibodies to tissue transglutaminase differentiate patients with dermatitis herpetiformis from those with linear IgA disease. J Am Acad Dermatol. 1999;41:957-61.

Sardy M, Karpati S, Merkl B, Paulsson M, Smyth N. Epidermal transglutaminase (TGase 3) is the autoantigen of dermatitis herpetiformis. J Exp Med. 2002;195:747-57.

Schmidt E, Zillikens D. Autoimmune and inherited subepidermal blistering diseases: advances in the clinic and the laboratory. Adv Dermatol. 2000;16:113-57.

Sontheimer RD, Provost TT, editors. Cutaneous manifestations of rheumatic diseases. Baltimore: Williams & Wilkins; 1996.

Stanley JR. Cell adhesion molecules as targets of autoantibodies in pemphigus and pemphigoid, bullous diseases due to defective epidermal cell adhesion. Adv Immunol. 1993;53:291-325.

Tan EM, Cohen AS, Fries JF, Masi AT, McShane DJ, Rothfield NF, et al. The 1982 revised criteria for the classification of systemic lupus erythematosus. Arthritis Rheum. 1982;25: 1271-7.

Vu TN, Lee TX, Ndoye A, Shultz LD, Pittelkow MR, Dahl MV, et al. The pathophysiological significance of non-desmoglein targets of pemphigus autoimmunity: development of antibodies against keratinocyte cholinergic receptors in patients with pemphigus vulgaris and pemphigus foliaceus. Arch Dermatol. 1998;134:971-80.

Woodley DT, Briggaman RA, O'Keefe EJ, Inman AO, Queen LL, Gammon WR. Identification of the skin basement-membrane autoantigen in epidermolysis bullosa acquisita. N Engl J Med. 1984;310:1007-13.

Zillikens D, Caux F, Mascaro JM, Wesselmann U, Schmidt E, Prost C, et al. Autoantibodies in lichen planus pemphigoides react with a novel epitope within the C-terminal NC16A domain of BP180. J Invest Dermatol. 1999;113:117-21.

Zillikens D, Rose PA, Balding SD, Liu Z, Olague-Marchan M, Diaz LA, et al. Tight clustering of extracellular BP180 epitopes recognized by bullous pemphigoid autoantibodies. J Invest Dermatol. 1997;109:573-9.

Zone JJ, Meyer LJ, Petersen MJ. Deposition of granular IgA relative to clinical lesions in dermatitis herpetiformis. Arch Dermatol. 1996;132:912-8.

Zone JJ, Taylor TB, Kadunce DP, Meyer LJ. Identification of the cutaneous basement membrane zone antigen and isolation of antibody in linear immunoglobulin A bullous dermatosis. J Clin Invest. 1990;85:812-20.

T - #0592 - 071024 - C88 - 279/216/4 - PB - 9780367390976 - Gloss Lamination